I0408859

35 Healthy Paleo and Keto Recipes

plus 31 Steps

to Lose weight with

Paleo Diet and a 7 Day

Keto Meal Plan

Paleo Diet for Beginners

31 Proven Steps to Lose Weight plus 23 Healthy Paleo Recipes

By Rebecca Publishing

Disclaimer

All the material contained in this book is provided for informational and educational purposes only. No responsibility can be taken for any outcomes resulting from the use of this material.

While every attempt has been made to provide information that is both accurate and effective, the author does not assume any responsibility for the accuracy or use/misuse of this information.

About the author!

I am a newbie to publishing business, but I have a lot of information to tell you. I have been studying healthy way of eating from leading nutritionist in Europe and I have a lot of useful information on this topic. I have lost more than 20 kilos so I can provide you with a lot of practical tips on this matter.

My story is also very bright, after giving birth to a child; I have gained a lot of extra weight. It was simply impossible to look into the mirror, but I decided to do my best to return to my previous shape. I have tried swimming, jogging, different diets like Dukan, Sugar Free Diet, Kremlyovskaya Diet etc. These diets forced me to starving and nothing more. I saw and fell the best result after following the Paleo Diet. This diet helped me to loose ALL my extra weight this is more than 20 kilos/44 pounds and I feel myself much healthier now! So, Let's start my explanation of what is it – paleo diet and the main aspects of it.

Introduction

Thank you for downloading of my book 31 Proven Steps to Loose Weight plus 23 Healthy Paleo Recipes. If you wish to loose weight and stay healthy, like people say, to kill two birds with one stone, then this book is the proper thing for you. So let`s begin our way to healthy life with beautiful body?

The History of Paleo Diet

I would like to tell you some words about the history of the Paleo Diet. This diet was developed and presented in the 1970s by the doctor, actually gastroenterologist. The name of this person is Walter Voegtlin. The main suggestion of him was to eat like our forefathers and become healthier, stronger and lean in such a way. What is more he claimed that this diet can reduce a lot of health problems such as diabetes, obesity and even Crohn`s disease. . It helps you to better your mental health. This diet is also a great way to make your face look better without spots and acne. What is more paleo diet makes a positive affect to your immune system as well as your digestion system. To crown it all the paleo diet can help you to minimize your blood pressure and better your sleep.

Mr Walter Voegtlin claimed, the main principles of this diet is to eat everything what our Paleolithic men consumed. These are mainly the following products: meats and fish (because it was easy to hunt for) also nuts, seeds, different fruits and vegetable. Everything is simple.

 Now I would like to proceed to the first chapter where I am going to list all 31 proven steps on paleo diet which will bring you to healthy way of living and beautiful shape.

35 Healthy Paleo and Keto Recipes plus 31 Steps to Lose weight with Paleo Diet and a 7 Day Keto Meal Plan

Chapter 1

31 Proven Steps of Paleo Diet for Beginners

1. You can replace sugar by the honey. This will add more vitamins into your daily menu and will not allow you to gain weight.

2. You can replace grains with all kinds of vegetables. You can eat them either fresh or frozen. Sweet potatoes and yams are allowed as well.

3. You can replace all sort of oils like corn oil or soy oil by home – made mayonnaise. Avoid eating fried food it affects destroying to your digestive organs.

4. Eat a lot of meat, it is better to eat meat from pastured animals. There are a lot of meat, which contains antibiotics; hormones try to avoid buying such sort of meat.

5. Try to include intake of eggs into your weekly rations, as eggs contain omega 3. You can enjoy different sorts of egg like: duck egg, chicken egg or goose egg.

6. Fish is also another useful thing into your daily menu, try to eat it at least two times per week.

7. Include fruits, but be aware that there is a lot of sugar in them, especially in tropical fruits, take you look mostly at berries. Fruits contain fructose which is not that good for the liver. But it is not that strict rule, so you can sometimes include apple, avocado, blackberries, peaches, plums, blueberries, lemon, watermelon, pineapple, oranges into your menu.

8. Try to include nuts into your daily menu, especially almonds, pistachios, cashews, hazelnuts etc.

9. Kefir, sour cream, different yogurts are allowed, they are very useful for the health in general.

10. It is better lower the intake of nuts, fruits to nearly 50 – 70 grams per day. If you wish to loose weight rapidly.

11. Eat if only you are hungry and every three hours.

12. Spare enough time for sleep it is better to make a regime for yourself, for instance sleep from ten pm till seven am the least.

13. Try to take not very hard exercise two times per week. Combine your exercise program, with daily rest.

14. Include vitamin D in your menu as it is one more important ingredient. Iodine is another important ingredient into your daily menu. You can take this vitamin from seaweeds, they are really reach for it.

15. You are free to eat leafy greens, like: spinach, iceberg lettuce, kale etc.

16. You can afford yourself even Dark Chocolate. It is necessary to find the dark chocolate of at least 70% - 80% cacao.

17. It is also possible to enjoy one glass of red wine per day.

18. You should drink at least one and a half liters of water per day.

19. It is necessary to mention some foods you should avoid to stay slim and healthy according to the rules of paleo diet. Natural carbs: Potatoes, Rice, milk , but dairy is allowed especially if you feel that it is necessary for your organs of digestion.

20. The most beautiful thing is that you do not have to limit your daily intake of food. But of course it is better to eat till the moment when you can feel that you are not hungry anymore, and not till when you are totally full.

21. Try to get outside to get sunshine as the more vitamin D you get the better for your health, but do not get burned!

22. Obtain a crock pot, as it is the best method to prepare paleo meals.

23. Do not hurry to see the results. Paleo diet is not a one day diet, it takes time, but it gives results as well.

24. Lower the intake of salt as it is not a good thing to your kidneys. It is worth mentioning, when you remove a lot of "negative foods" from your menu you will understand that it is totally ok to eat without salt and sugar, or cook with the help of crock pot and the food tastes better, much better.

25. You can enjoy of all sort of animal organs like: tongue, kidney liver and marrow.

26. You can also enjoy eating different sea food things like: shrimps, scallops, herring, shark and much more.

27. It is also allowed to include different sorts of mushrooms. They are totally allowed.

28. You can use a lot of substitution to feel yourself satisfied with what you it, there are some of them listed below:
    - Sea salt instead of iodized salt.
    - Homemade paleo bread, instead of bread you can buy at the market.
    - Cauliflower instead of rice and potatoes.

29. Remember! All sorts of fruit juices are also very rich in fructose so it is better to stay away from them. These are

- Apple juice
- Orange juice
- Grape juice
- Strawberry juice
- Mango juice

30. It is also necessary to stay away from snacks. These are all sorts of chips, cookies, different pastries etc.

31. Also remove alcohol and energy drink from your list if you wish to stay healthy and lose your extra weight.

Chapter 2

IN THIS CHAPTER I WOULD LIKE TO GIVE YOU A VERY IMPORTANT INFORMATION AS FOR YOUR DAILY MENU, WHICH WILL HELP YOU TO START YOUR PALEO DIET EASILY. SO LETS BEGIN

For breakfast:

The best and the healthiest thing will be omelet with some onion, broccoli or mushrooms. You can also add chicken or turkey.

For Lunch:

The best thing is to prepare a big bowl with vegetables like radish, spinach, cucumbers, carrot, you can also add almonds or walnuts. You are welcome to add such sorts of meat as chicken, turkey, beef to your plate or you can add something from fish like shrimp, tuna, salmon etc.

For Dinner:

It is possible to make a spaghetti squash instead of pasta recipe with meatballs, or also different sorts of seafood or fresh food with broccoli, or vegetables a great idea for paleo dinner.

You can take berries for your dessert

35 Healthy Paleo and Keto Recipes plus 31 Steps to Lose weight with Paleo Diet and a 7 Day Keto Meal Plan

Bonus Chapter 3

15 yummy paleo recipes for every day.

Breakfast recipes:

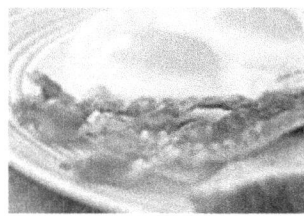

1.Becon and egg Paradise

Ingredients:

3 - 6 eggs

3 slices of cut bacon

2 cups of spinach chopped

A bit of salt and pepper

Instructions:

Heat your oven to 350F

Mix the eggs in a bowl

Cook the becon in a skillet

Add a spinach to this skillet and cook for 10 more minutes

Add eggs into this skillet and add a bit of salt and pepper.

Bake for 15 more minutes

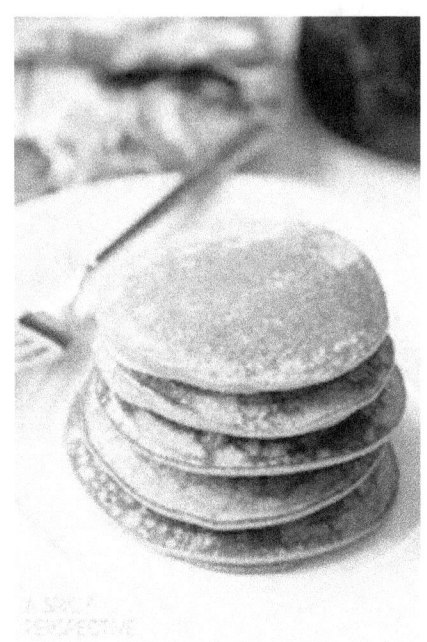

2. Perfect Paleo Pancakes (nut-free)

Ingredients:

4 Eggs

Half of a cup of coconut flour

1table spoon of honey

1 table spoon of vinegar

a half of a spoon of baking soda

a bit of a salt

1 table spoon of vanilla

Instructuions:

1. Put all the dry pancake ingredients in a bowl. Whip in all the liquid ingredients (do not add the coconut milk).

2. Gradually add the coconut milk. You will need to add as much coconut milk as you need until you see the preferable consistency.

3. Preheat a consistency and coat with grease with coconut oil.

4. Pour a spoon of a pancake batter onto the griddle. Make the pancakes about 3-4 inches in diameter as it will be easier to operate them. Bake for 2-3 minutes, then turn them on another side for an additional 1-2 minutes.

5. Take away from a pan and serve with your chosen syrup.

6. Enjoy your breakfast.

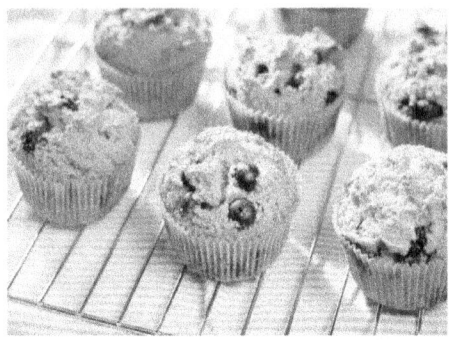

3. Paleo Blueberry Muffin

Ingredients:

1 cup of almond flour

A bit of soda

A bit of salt on your taste

1 egg

2 tbsp of honey

A half of a cup of fresh blueberries

A half of a cup of coconut milk

2 tbsp of coconut oil

Instructions:

1. Heat the oven to 350°F.

2. Mix all together salt, baking soda and almond flour

3. Whip all together the honey, coconut milk, coconut oil, and egg.

4. Then mix the wet and the dry ingredients together, but not that much.

5. Add blueberries into the dough.

6. Add the prepared dough into the muffin tin and bake

7. Bake until a toothpick inserted into the center comes out clean, about 20-25 minutes

8. Set pan over a wire rack to cool. Wait until muffins are completely cool before removing from the paper liners.

9. Recipe makes 6 muffins. Store in an airtight container in the refrigerator.

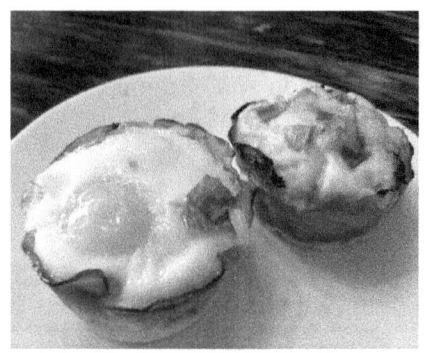

4. Paleo Breakfast: Baked Eggs in Ham Cups

Ingredients:

Eggs

Ham or Turkey

Instructions:

1. Heat the oven to 400°F.
2. Grease your muffin pan.
3. Slice the ham and put it into the muffin cup, one or two slices is enough for each cup.
4. You can scramble your eggs or even whip them or you can just put the whole egg into the muffin cup. (Optional) If you do wish to make scrambled eggs you can also add there different ingredients, like mushrooms, onion, different greens and spinach.
5. Preheat the oven ti 400°F , put the muffin pan in to the oven and bake for 15 – 20 more minutes

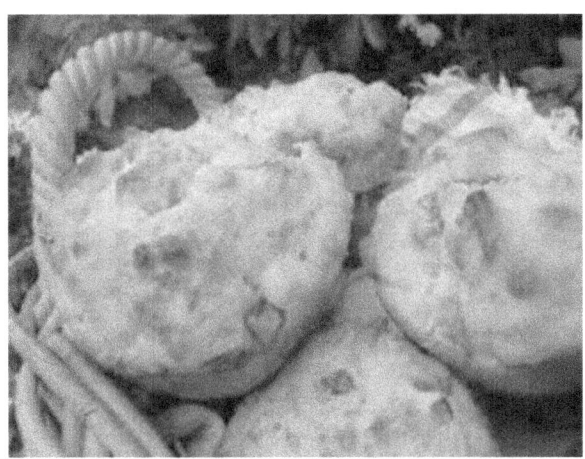

5. Avocado & Bacon Muffins

Ingredients:

1 onion

4 eggs

6 -7 slices of bacon

2 cups avocado

one and a half of a cup of coconut flour

a half of a tea spoon of baking soda

salt & pepper

1 cup of coconut milk

Instructions:

1.Heat the oven to 175 degrees Celsius (350F)

2.Grease 12 muffin pans with oil. (melt it before)

3.Finely chop onion and bacon.

4.Brown in a fry pan.

5.Mix the avocado and eggs very good.

6.Stir in the milk.

7.Add coconut flour, salt, pepper and baking soda and stir it all well

8.Fold through three quarters of the cooked bacon and onion mixture.

9.Put this into the muffin pans.

10.Put on the top bacon and onion.

11.Bake in the oven for approximately 20 25 minutes.

12.Cool before taking the muffins out.

13.Enjoy your breakfast.

LUNCH RECIPES

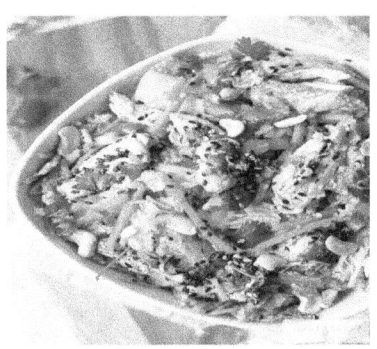

6.Super Paleo Chinese Chicken Salad

Ingredients:

1 carrot

1 large Napa Cabbage, it is necessary to chop it into slices.

1 chicken, sliced into thin peaces.

A half of a cup chopped cilantro

2 tablespoons of black sesame seeds and 2 table spoons of white sesame seeds

1/4 cup of gluten free soy sauce, I prefer Tamari.

1/4 cup white wine vinegar

3 table spoons of a minced ginger

3 table spoons of olive oil

1 table spoon of toasted sesame oil

1 table spoon of Spicy Chili Oil

Some sea salt on your taste

Some chopped green onions

For the dressing:

In a small bowl with lid add tamari sauce, vinegar, olive oil, hoisin sauce, toasted sesame oil, chili oil, sriracha, minced ginger, sea salt and chopped green onions. Shake it all together. Set aside. Then add, chopped cabbage, sliced carrot, cilantro, sesame seeds, cashews, sliced chicken, and dressing into a large plastic bowl, shake until well enough. Add more dressing if needed.

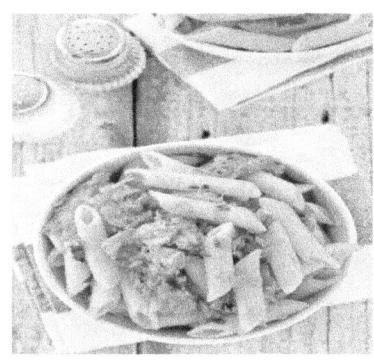

7.Spicy Tuna and Tomato

Ingredients:

1 cup of tuna

1 red onion, chopped

1 small red chilli, chopped as well

1 peace of garlic

1 egg

2 Tbsp of tomato paste

1 Tbsp of coconut flour

Salt and pepper on your taste

You can also add:

Lettuce

Avocado

Extra chilli, if you wish it to be hot

35 Healthy Paleo and Keto Recipes plus 31 Steps to Lose weight with Paleo Diet and a 7 Day Keto Meal Plan

Instructions:

1 – Pre-heat your oven to 350'F

2 – Put a parchment paper on a baking tray and set aside for now.

3 – Put all the burger ingredients into a bowl and stir all them well

4. Make with your hands bolls using this tuna mixture. Place all of them into the baking sheet

5 – Place in the oven and cook approximately for 5-10 mins, until they are cooked enough.

6 – To serve, place these cute balls on a lettuce leaf (or 2) put some fresh sliced avocado on top, and sprinkle over some fresh coriander and some slices of chilli.

Enjoy your meal!

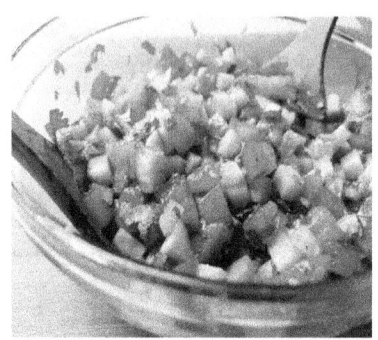

8.Cucumber and Tomato Salad

Ingredients:

one clove Garlic

one cup of Olives

one tablespoon of fresh Basil, (it is necessary to slice it very thin)

one table spoon of Fresh Oregano, (it is necessary to chop it)

two cups of Cucumber, sliced or chopped.

Two cups of Grape Tomatoes

Two table spoons of Balsamic Vinegar

Two table spoons of Extra Virgin Olive Oil

One table spoon of Black Pepper

Instructions:

1. Rinse, then slice or chop your cucumbers.

2. Rinse grape tomatoes, cut them in half.

3. Thinly slice basil, cut oregano, mince garlic.

4. Mix everything with the kalamata olives in a bowl, sprinkle with olive oil and balsamic vinegar, and add a bit of black pepper.

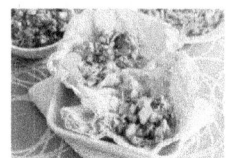

9.Chicken and avocado Lettuce Wraps

Ingredients:

One cup cooked and sliced Chicken, Boneless Breasts

One and a half cup of mashed avocado, peel the coat before mashing.
one tbsp. of juice Lemon

one tbsp. of juice Lime

two tbsp. of Yogurt

two tbsp of choped Cilantro

Salt on your taste

Black Pepper on your taste

Serving Day Ingredients

One cup of grape tomatoes

Instructions:

1. Chop chicken breast

2. Mash avocado, lemon juice, lime juice, and yogurt in a bowl and stir well, until it becomes creamy!

3. Add salt, pepper and cilantro to the chopped chicken, according to your taste.

4. Spoon into lettuce wraps, put tomatoes on top, and serve.

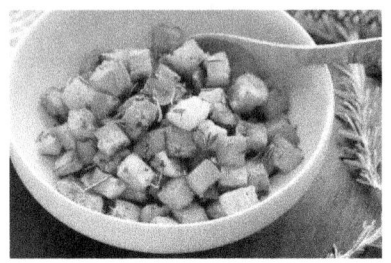

10. Sweet Potato

Ingredients:

2 Medium sweet potatoes chopped into small cubes

3 tbsp of coconut oil

Sea salt

Instructions:

1. Boil water in a medium pot
2. Chop sweet potato into cubes
3. Put the sweet potato into the boiling water for around five minutes and take It away when it becomes slightly softened.
4. Drain and dry the sweet potatoes
5. Heat up the coconut oil in the large skillet, make the heat medium.

6. Toss in the sweet potatoes cubes and let them cook well for approximately six or seven minutes. Continue doing it until they are nice and brown. Sprinkle with sea salt according to your taste. Your sweet potatoes will be yummy, crispy and goldy brown if you let them cook well enough.

ENJOY YOUR MEAL!

DINNER RECIPES

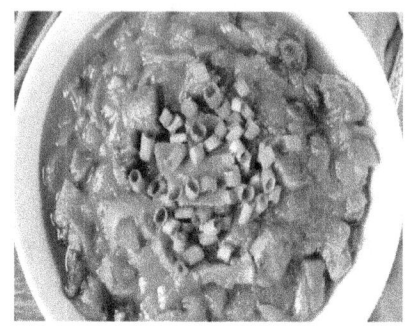

11.Paleo Pizza Soup

Ingredients:

10-12 chicken sausage, slice them

4 – 5 uncured pepperoni,

5-7 roasted tomatoes

1 medium size onion,

10-15 mushrooms, slice them

1 can of black olives, slice them

1 tbsp of dried oregano

1 tsp of garlic powder

Salt to taste

Instructions:

1. Put the sausage, pepperoni, marinara, tomatoes, onion, mushrooms, olives, oregano, garlic powder, and salt into the pan

2. Cook for about 30 minutes. It is considered to be ready when onions and mushrooms have softened.

3. Add more salt if needed.

4. Serve hot.

5. Enjoy this delicious meal.

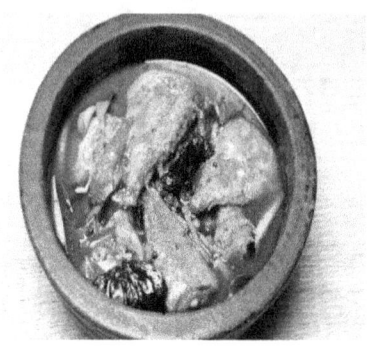

12.Quick and Easy Fish Curry

Ingredients:

2 Tbsp of coconut oil

1 onion,

3 cloves of garlic, chopped or mashed

2 Tbsp of ginger

2 tsp of curry powder

10 - 15 curry leaves

400ml of coconut milk

2 tomatoes, chopp them

Sea salt on your taste

600g of white fish, cut into peaces

Juice of a lime on your taste

Large handful leaves of coriander

Instructions:

1. Melt the coconut oil in the pan.

2. Add sliced onion there and make it brown

3. Than add the garlic and ginger and cook for approximately one minute.

4. Add the turmeric, curry leaves and do not forget about the curry powder.

5. Continue to cook during one minute, then gradually stir in the coconut milk.

6. Simmer it.

7. Add the chopped tomato and simmer for additional five minutes until the tomato become soft.

8. Add the fish, add some salt on your taste and wait until the fish is cooked.

9. Add coriander and lime juice and stir it all well.

10. It is a very delicious with rice

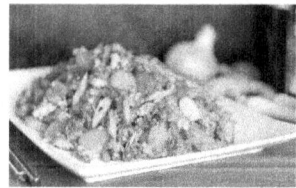

13.Paleo Pineapple Fried Rice

Ingredients:

Three table spoons of avocado oil

two cups of fresh pineapple, cut for the slices

one red bell pepper

four small carrots

two cloves garlic, minced

a bit of green onions, thinly sliced

four eggs

Sauce:

¼ cup coconut aminos

2 tsp of chili paste

As a final step:

one cup of roasted cashew pieces

Sea salt on your taste

Instructions:

1. Prepare all your ingredients, wash and cut them

2. Take away the core with its seeds from the bell pepper and cut it thoroughly.

3. Peel the carrots and cut it into cubes.

4. Grate the cauliflower.

5. Crack the eggs into a plastic bowl and mix them with the fork or whatever.

6. Put together the coconut aminos and chili paste in a bowl and set it aside.

7. After you have prepared everything, preheat your pan

8. Add one tbsp of the avocado oil to the frying pan and also add the pineapple chunks to create the tasty and caramelized edges. Then take away the pineapples and put it into the separate bowl, until you prepare the rice. After add the green onions and cauliflower. It is necessary to cook it for about several minutes to make the cauliflower soft.

9. Then add all the veggies into the pan; pepper, garlic, carrots and make them crispy.

10. Add the sauce to the pan and let it to prepare for several more minutes until the sauce is gone and mix everything well.

11. Take away the fried rice from the heat and join it to cashews and caramelized pineapple. Add some sea salt if necessary.

12.It tastes simply amazing both hot and taken from the refrigerator.

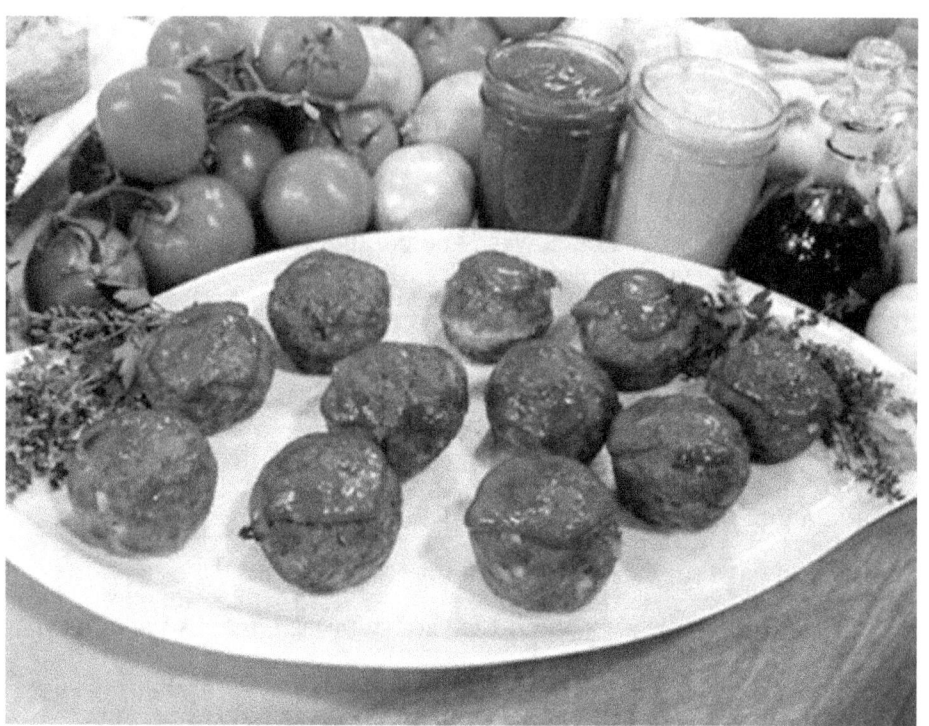

14.Paleo Mini Meatloaves

Ingredients:

two pounds of meat – it is better to mix beef with pork or veal

chopped spinach, the amount on your preference

one or two teaspoons oil

one medium onion,

ten - fifteen mushrooms, finely diced

two grated carrots,

four eggs,

1/3 cup coconut flour

two tsp of salt

two tsp of pepper

two tsp of onion powder

one tsp of garlic powder

one tsp of dried thyme and a bit of grated nutmeg.

Instructions:

1. Preheat oven to **375 degrees F**

2. Prepare spinach and set aside.

3. Preheat a pan add the oil and add there onions, mushrooms. Cook everything until the onion become translucent and some water is gone. Than you can set this pan aside. Place the ground meat in a large bowl, add the spinach, carrots, mushroom/onion mixture, beaten eggs, coconut flour and all the spices. Mix everything, but not that much, just to make all the ingredients well – organized.

4. Add this mixture into muffin tins. It is better to grease the tins.

5. Cook for 20-25 minutes until total preparation.

6. This dish is better to serve hot.

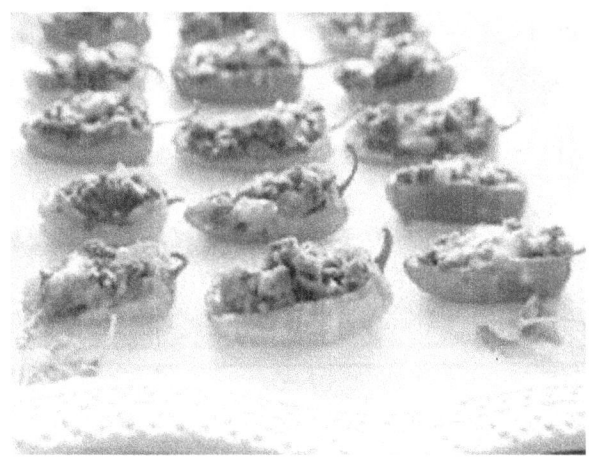

15. Stuffed Baby Sweet Peppers

Ingredients:

Fifteen - twenty mini sweet peppers

Six ounces of goat cheese

A half of a cup of ricotta cheese

One tea spoon of garlic powder

A bit of pepper powder

Salt to your taste

Instructions:

1. Preheat oven to 375F. Lean baking sheet with foil.

2. Wash the peppers and cut in half lengthwise. Remove all the seeds

3. Than mash together the goat cheese, the ricotta, and the seasonings well.

4. Snip the corner off of a small ziploc bag and put cheese mixture into this bag. Squeeze the bag and pipe the cheese into the pepper halves.

5. Put the peppers on the baking sheet and cook it for about 5-6 minutes until nicely browned. It is possible to prepare this delicious thing on the grill as well.

6. Enjoy!

Some more Paleo Recipes

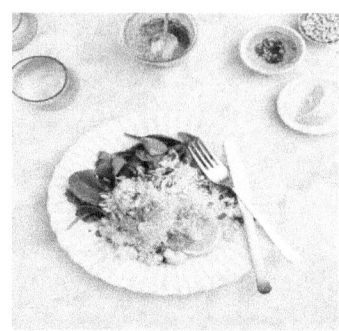

16. Creamy Lemon Basil Spaghetti Squash

Ingredients:

One Avocado (a half of a cup mashed)

six garlic cloves

one cup fresh basil leaves

one tbsp lemon zest

one third of a cup lemon juice

two tbsp. of olive oil

if you wish you can add cayenne pepper on your taste

a half of tsp black pepper

a sea salt on your taste

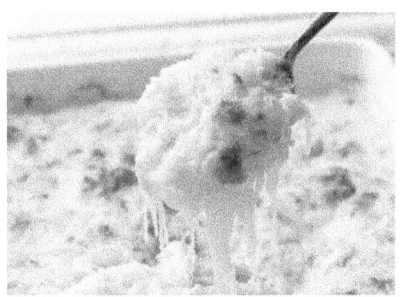

17. Spaghetti Squash
Ingredients:

1. two tsp olive oil
2. three cups spaghetti squash, cooked
3. one cup of chopped kale
4. 10-15 cherry tomatoes
5. A half of tsp black pepper
6. sea salt on your taste

Instructions:

1. Mix all the sauce ingredients into blender. Puree them thoroughly
2. Heat the pan and add the olive oil. When the oil is hot add the tomatoes and sauté about two minutes.
3. Add the other ingredients and sauté approximately five minutes. Add about a half of a cup of the sauce and mix thoroughly.
4. Bon appetite!!!

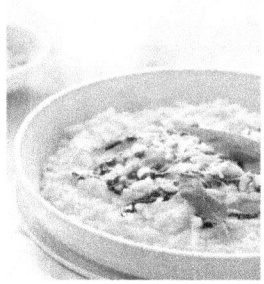

18. Butternut Squash Risotto

Ingredients:

1½ pounds butternut squash, peeled and cubed (about 4 cups)

1 tablespoon solid cooking fat

½ yellow onion, chopped

1 cup mushrooms, chopped

3 cloves garlic, minced

¼ cup sage, minced

½ teaspoon sea salt

1 teaspoon apple cider vinegar

¾ cup bone broth

Instructions:

1. Place half of the chopped butternut squash into a food processor and pulse for 20 seconds, until the squash is the consistency of rice. Don't over process here!

2. Heat the solid cooking fat in the bottom of a large skillet or heavy-bottomed pot on medium heat. When the fat has melted and the pan is hot, add the onions and

mushrooms. Cook, stirring, until the onions are translucent, about 5 minutes. Add the garlic, sage, and sea salt, and cook for another 2 minutes, just until fragrant.

3. Add the apple cider vinegar and scrape away anything that has stuck to the bottom of the pan. Add the processed squash and bone broth to the pan, stirring to incorporate. Cook for 12-15 minutes on medium heat uncovered, stirring occasionally, until the liquid has absorbed and the squash is fully cooked.

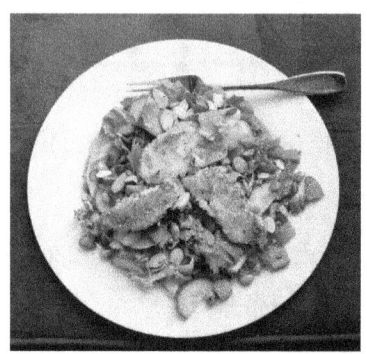

19. Coconut Crusted Chicken Salad

Ingredients:

2 tbsp Coconut flour

2 tbsp Unsweetened flaked coconut

2 Chicken fillets

1 Egg (beaten)

2 cups Spring mix salad greens

3 tbsp Apple cider vinegar

1 tsp Honey

3 tbsp olive oil

2 tbsp Coconut oil

Salt and pepper (to taste)

Instructions:

1. Create a breading/dredging station with three plates or shallow bowls.

2. Add the coconut flour to one, the the egg to the second plate and the flaked coconut to the third.

3. Heat the coconut oil in a skillet over medium-high heat.

4. Dredge each chicken fillet in the coconut flour first, followed by the egg, coating each evenly. Then the flaked coconut. Be sure the fillet is coated well.

5. Place each fillet into the hot skillet. Cook on each side, about 5 minutes. Until the chicken is golden in color and cooked through.

6. Add the apple cider vinegar and honey to a bowl. Whisk to combine. Continue to whisk while drizzling in the olive oil until well combined and becomes creamy. Season with salt and pepper.

7. Place the spring mix in a mixing bowl. Drizzle the dressing over and toss to coat. Reserve ½ to serving.

8. Plate the spring mix evenly then serve the chicken on top. Serve with additional dressing on the side. Season with salt and pepper, to taste.

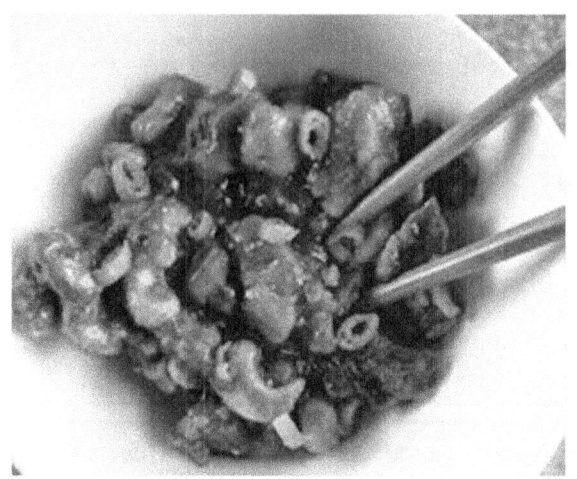

20. Paleo Crock Pot Cashew Chicken

Ingredients:

1/4 cup arrowroot starch

1/2 tsp. black pepper

2 lbs. chicken thighs, cut into bite-size pieces

1 tbs. coconut oil

3 tbs. coconut aminos

2 tbs. rice wine vinegar

2 tbs. organic ketchup (tomato paste would work also)

1/2-1 tbs. palm sugar

2 minced garlic cloves

1/2 tsp. minced fresh ginger

1/4-1/2 red pepper flakes

1/2 cup raw cashews

Instructions:

Place starch and black pepper in a large Ziploc bag. Add chicken pieces and seal; toss to thoroughly coat meat.

Melt coconut oil in a large skillet or wok. Add chicken and cook for about 5 minutes until brown on all sides. Remove and add to crock pot.

Mix coconut aminos through red pepper flakes in a small bowl. Pour mixture over chicken and toss to coat. Put lid on crock pot and cook on low for 3-4 hours.

Stir cashews into chicken and sauce before serving.

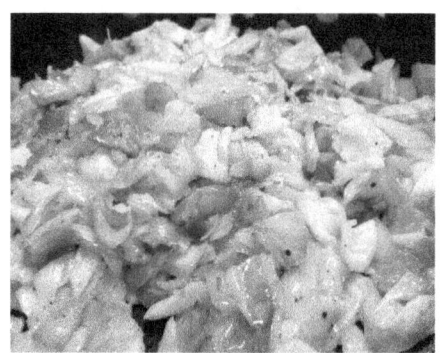

21. Fried Cabbage with Bacon, Onion, and Garlic

Ingredients:

Six slices of chopped becon

one large onion

two cloves of garlic

One cabbage

Salt on your taste

Pepper on your taste

A half of a teaspoon of onion powder

A half of a tea spoon of garlic powder

Instructions:

1. Put the bacon in a large stockpot and cook it until it becomes crispy. It should take you about ten minutes. Add the garlic and onion. cook until the onion caramelizes; about ten minutes. Then Stir in the cabbage and continue to cook and stir for another 10 minutes. Add salt, pepper, onion powder, paprika and garlic powder. After all simmer for about 30 minutes more.

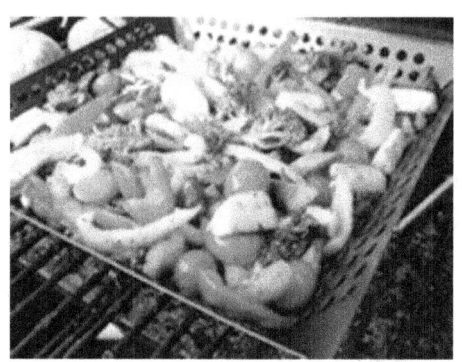

22. Roasted Tasty Vegetable Medley

Ingredients:

2 tbsp olive oil

One yam, peeled and cut into pieces.

One parsnip, peeled and cut into pieces.

One carrot

One zucchini, cut into pieces

One bunch of a fresh asparagus, also cut into pieces

Two cloves of a minced garlic

Fresh basil, on your taste

Pepper on your taste

Instructions:

1. Heat the oven and grease the baking sheet with olive oil.
2. Put the yams, parsnips, and carrots onto the baking sheets. Bake in the oven for 30 minutes, after put the zucchini and asparagus, and sprinkle with the 1 tablespoon of olive oil. Proceed baking until all of the vegetables are cooked, about 30 minutes more. Then remove from the oven, and allow to cool.
3. Toss the roasted peppers with the garlic, basil, salt, and pepper in a large bowl. Add the roasted vegetables, and mix everything well.

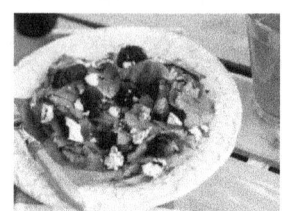

23. Delicious Beet Greens

Ingredients:

Two bunches beet greens

One table spoon of olive oil

Two cloves of garlic minced

Red pepper on your taste

Salt and pepper on your taste

Two lemons, cut into four slices

Instructions:

1. Put water into a pot let it to boil and salt it. Add the beet greens and cook them until they become tender. It will take you about two minutes. Drain beet greens then immerse with the ice water.

2. Bring a large pot of lightly salted water to a boil. Add the beet greens, and cook uncovered until tender, about 2 minutes. Drain in a colander, then immediately immerse in ice water for several minutes. Then chop the greens.

3. Heat the olive oil. Stir in the garlic and red pepper; cook and stir for one minute. Add salt and pepper. Cook until greens are hot; serve with lemon.

Thank You

I am very happy that you have chosen this book and it's been a real pleasure writing it for you. My aim is to help as many readers as possible. So many of us are able to take new knowledge and use it to our lives with really useful and long lasting consequences and it is my desire that you have been able to take value from the information I have written.

Thank you for beeing with me during this book and for reading it through to the end. I really hope that you have enjoyed the information and that's why I appreciate your thoughts on my material so much. If you could take a couple of minutes to write a feedback, your views will help me to create more material that you find beneficial.

Thanks again for your attention. I really look forward to reading your review.

Stay Healthy!

KETOGENIC DIET FOR BEGINNERS

12 SUPER EASY KETO RECIPES

AND A 7 DAY MEAL PLAN

By Rebecca Publishing

Disclaimer

All the material contained in this book is provided for informational and educational purposes only. No responsibility can be taken for any outcomes resulting from the use of this material.

While every attempt has been made to provide information that is both accurate and effective, the author does not assume any responsibility for the accuracy or use/misuse of this information.

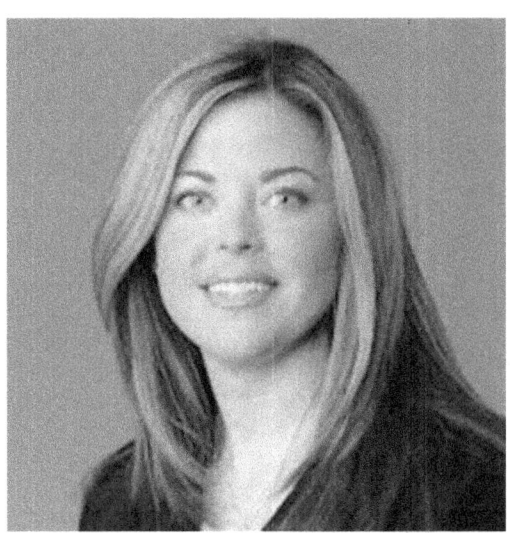

About the author!

I am a newbie to publishing business, but I have a lot of information to tell you. I have been studying healthy way of eating from leading nutritionist in Europe and I have a lot of useful information concerning this topic. I have lost more than 20 kilos so I can provide you with a lot of practical tips on this matter.

My story is also very bright, after giving birth to a child; I gained a lot of extra weight. It was simply impossible to look into the mirror, but I decided to do my best to return myself to my previous shape. I have tried swimming, jogging, different diets like Dukan, Sugar Free Diet, Kremlyovskaya Diet etc. These diets forced me to starving and nothing more. I saw and fell the best result after following the Paleo Diet combined with Ketogenic Diet. This diet helped me to loose ALL my extra weight this is more than 20 kilos/44 pounds and

I feel myself much healthier now! I would like to provide you with detailed information about Ketogenic Diet in this book.

Introduction

Thank you for downloading of my book 31 Proven Steps to Lose Weight plus 23 Healthy Paleo Recipes. If you wish to become slimmer and stay healthy, like people say, to kill two birds with one stone, then this book is the proper thing for you. So let`s begin our way to healthy life with beautiful body?

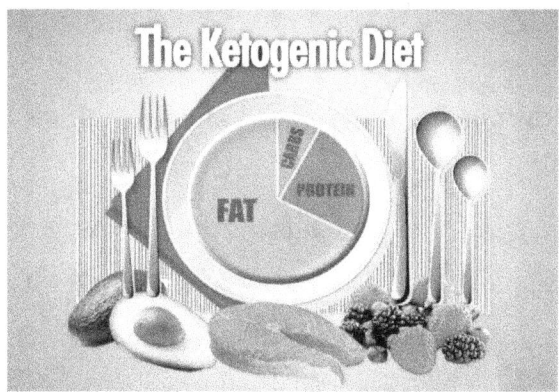

Ketogenic Diet

Eager to be well-turned but not tormented by hunger? Note the Keto Diet! Its unique principles designed just for you! It promises you to break yourself of extra kilos as fast as it possible! Furthermore, you wouldn't suffer from starvation for months. Forget about calories and portions. A Ketogenic Diet is of great mark and mysterious diet for excess weight tired humanity!

HISTORICAL INFORMATION

Keto Diet is not a fashionable novelty. This diet restricts carbohydrates and gives the "green light" fats. First eating plan was evolved by Dr. Russell Wilder at the Mayo Clinic to lend a helping hand children who suffer from epilepsy seizures. It has been clinically tested in the beginning of XX century. During the 1920s-1930s it got popular thanks to its effectiveness, but   in the 40-ies - treatment of epileptic attacks by medication became more widespread thus and so the Ketogenic Diet was dead as dodo.

The situation has improved in recent years. The Ketogenic Diet is becoming increasingly popular. What is behind everybody's interest in this diet? People were tired of being fat! This moment humanity was mad about highly powerful method of losing body weight (particularly, losing fat). Quite a number of people have found that this mysterious diet helps them to be rosy about the gills and keep fit. It helped many human beings to work off excess weight, improve health, and to be full of pith.

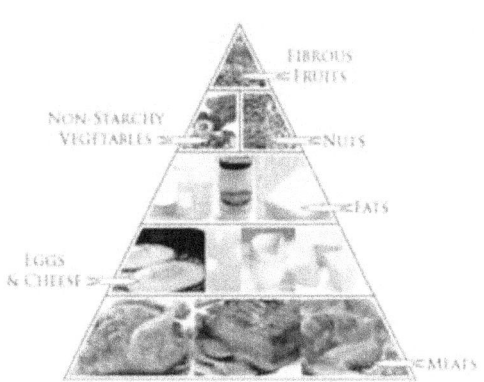

What is a Keto or Ketogenic Diet?

The Ketogenic Diet (or Keto) is a very low-carbohydrate, high-fat diet.

Here are ultimate diet tenets

•   Eat food which is poor in carbohydrates.

•   Eat plenty of fats.

•   Have food with a moderate rate of proteins.

Keto-diet bears resemblance to other low-carbohydrate diets. But it is more limited than for example the Atkins diet where you can take any kind of fat. It makes your body to destroy fatty cells (in a form of ketones - bodies, formed as a consequence of fat metabolism) rather than sugar (in a type of glucose/glycogen). This process involves radically reducing carbs consumption, and substituting it with fat. Sharp decrease in carbs brings human organism into a metabolic state which is called ketosis.

69

Usually for these purposes body needs carbohydrates, but in case of their lack, the body finds a solution and resorts to the fats. They are becoming the principal source of energy. Body also transforms fatty cells into ketones in the liver, which can give your brain extra boost.

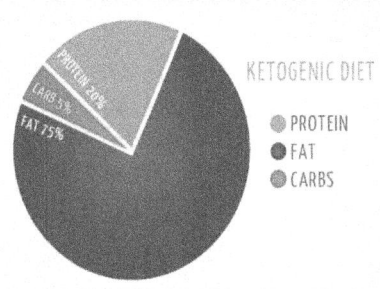

Health Benefits of the Ketogenic Diet

Proven for use that low-cabs diet has a beneficial effect on human health:

• Heart disease: improves risk coefficients like body fat depositions, tension of blood and blood-sugar levels, HDL levels.

• Epilepsy: having recurrence to the diet it is possible to lower the percentage of epileptic attacks in kids

• Cancer: helps to maintain the body of the patients, in a few isolated instances treats varieties of cancer and raises index of tumor growth inhibition.

• Alzheimer's disease: the diet greatly relieves symptoms of the disease and brakes down progressive illness.

• Parkinson's disease: as a consequence of taking low-carb, patients suffering from Parkinson's disease feel better

71

•   Polycystic ovary syndrome: diet menu plan declines insulin levels that is vitally important for patients.

•   Brain injuries: reduces severe concussions of the brain and raises prospect of recovery after cerebral damages.

Choose your Ketogenic Diet!

Pay attention to four varieties of Keto Diet

1)Standard ketogenic diet (SKD): its concept - more fats (around 75%), 20% proteins and 5% carbohydrates.

2)Cyclical ketogenic diet (CKD): alternation of food - five keto-days then two high-carbohydrates.

3)Targeted ketogenic diet (TKD): add carbohydrates around exercise conditioning.

4)High-protein ketogenic diet: duplicate SKD, but requires some more protein. Its tenets - 60% fats, more proteins (around 35%) and 5% carbs.

BUT Only first and fourth kinds of keto-diet are under active consideration. The 2-nd and the 3-d diets - more improved techniques, and mainly musclemen or athletes adhere to its rules.

REMEMBER If you take a Keto-Diet, you shouldn't go beyond the limit of carbs under 30g.

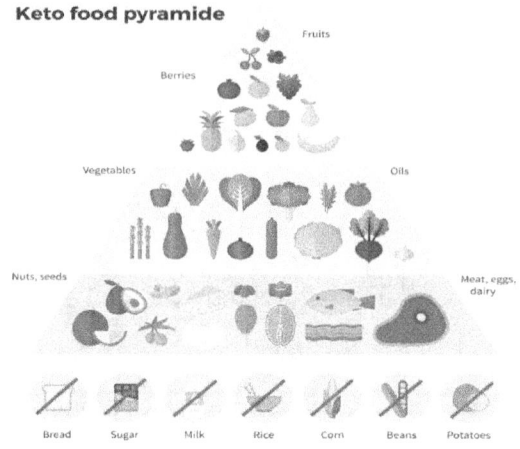

What color of food do you prefer?

Green food - Great: more fats (polyunsaturated or saturated), less carbs.

Blue food - Good: moderate amount of fats, less carbohydrates.

Orange food - Permissible: high fats and moderate quantity of carbs

Red food - Barely permissible: less fats, more carbohydrates.

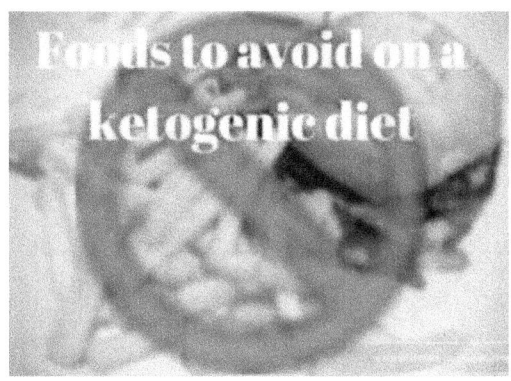

Foods to Avoid

Avoid any factory-farmed meat, food that is rich in carbohydrates, and processed foods.

• Sugary foods: in any form (solid and liquid). This is the main enemy. sugary soft-drinks, candy bars, chocolate, cake, ice cream, candy, fruit juices, table sugar and all items that have extra sugar in them.

• All grains or starches: grain products (loaf bread, any pizza, cookies, buns, crackers), wheat-based food products, barley, rye.

• Dairy products: All the milk-containing product should be avoided. Only a few sips of full-fat, raw milk is allowed. Why milk and dairy products? Milk is poorly digested and it is quite high in carbohydrates (four-five grams of carbohydrates per 100 ml). If you like coffee and tea with milk, replace it with good cream in permissible amounts.

• Fruit: tropical fruits such as pineapples, , bananas, papaya, mangoes etc. and forbidden high-carbohydrate fruits (tangerines, grapes).

• Beans or legumes: lentils, beans, chickpeas, peas, etc.

- Unhealthy fat: refined fats / oils - sunflower oil, soya bean oil, mayonnaise, olive oil, margarine, corn oil.

- Roots and tubers: carrots, potatoes, beat, parsnips, etc.

- Some condiments or sauces: contain sugar and unhealthy fat.

- Alcohol: beer, sweet wine etc. Alcoholic beverages contain a lot of extra calories.

- Low-fat or health food: may be often high in carbohydrates or include gluten, artificial additives, etc

Foods to Eat

Base the majority of your meals around these foods and eat freely:

- Meat: lamb, ham, sausage, beef, turkey, chicken, goat, mutton,

- Seafood, fish: fatty fish (salmon, trout, tuna).

- Eggs: take eggs enriched with Omega 3.

- Butter and cream: use grass-fed when possible.

- Nuts and seeds: almonds, pumpkin seeds, walnuts etc.

- Greengrocery and vegetables: avocados, law-carbohydrate vegetables such as peppers, onions, tomatoes, broccolis.

- Beverages and Condiments: still water, coffee (black or with coconut milk or cream), black or herbal tea, homemade condiments (mayonnaise, mustard, pesto) with no additives, garlic, pepper, high quality sea salt and various safe spices and herbs.

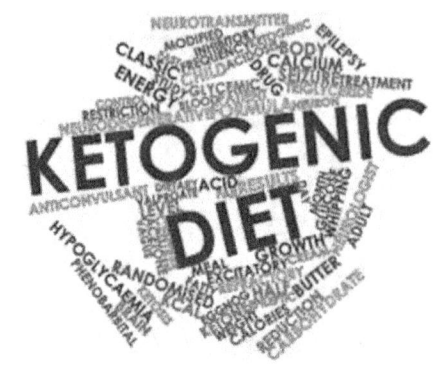

The Ketogenic Diet 7-day menu plan

1st Day – Monday

Breakfast: 2 fried eggs (use coconut oil) and steamed vegetables. One apple or any greengrocery you like.

Lunch: 2 or 3 nuts. Take a chicken salad with an olive oil.

Dinner: Two burgers (if you like) fried in butter and few boiled vegetables or choose salsa.

2nd Day – Tuesday

Breakfast: Have any allowed fruit. 2 eggs with bacon.

Lunch: Two burgers (if you like) that are fried in butter and boil two or more vegetables. Have a fruit mix salad?

Dinner: Fried fatty salmon (use butter). Vegetable mix salad.

3d Day – Wednesday

Breakfast: Chicken, beet, pork or anything meat you like and boiled (steamed) vegetables.

Lunch: Sandwich with a leaf of lettuce; boiled chicken with boiled vegetables.

Dinner: Some berries or nuts, fried beef, grilled vegetables.

4th Day – Thursday

Breakfast: Fried eggs and any low-carbs fruit.

Lunch: Have three or four nuts, a piece of boiled chicken and mixed vegetables.

Dinner: Boiled vegetables and baked meat.

5th Day – Friday

Breakfast: Fried chicken eggs (use coconut oil). and green foods.

Lunch: Some nuts. Chicken salad with an olive oil

Dinner: Take one juicy beef steak with fresh green vegetables and sweet potato for desert.

6th Day – Saturday

Breakfast: Any fresh fruit you like. Eggs with bacon.

Lunch: One beef steak with steamed (or grilled) vegetables.

Dinner: Salmon that is baked in olive oil. One tropic fruit (eg. avocado) and raw vegetables too.

7th Day – Sunday

Breakfast: Boiled carrot, beet etc. and turkey or goat.

Lunch: One sandwich, boiled chicken and fresh raw vegetables salad.

Dinner: Roasted chicken wings (you'd better to use olive oil) combined with boiled vegetables.

Do you believe that you can eat a lot of fatty, delicious and full meal? And at mealtime you lose weight and large volumes? Perhaps this diet is the dream path to the perfect figure!

RECIPES OF DISHES FOR KETO-DIET BREAKFAST (LUNCH)

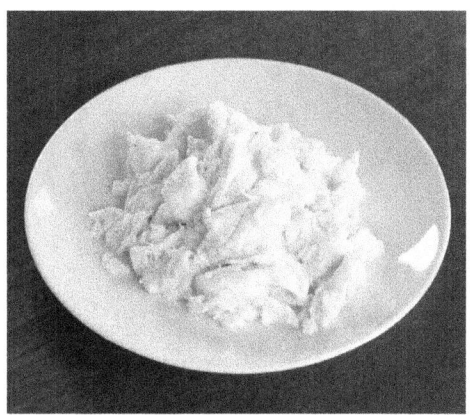

1. Scrambled Eggs

INGREDIENTS

Fresh hen eggs - 3 pcs

Unsalted butter - 1 tblsp.

Salt, pepper

METHOD OF PREPARATION

1. Beat up eggs (better with a fork).

2. Soften the butter.

3. Combine egg mass with butter.

4. Empty out this mass into the hot pan.

5. Cook eggs during 60 seconds on one side and then quickly move and cook during one minute on the other side.

6. Scrambled eggs are ready!

7. Put some salt and black pepper!

8. Enjoy hot!

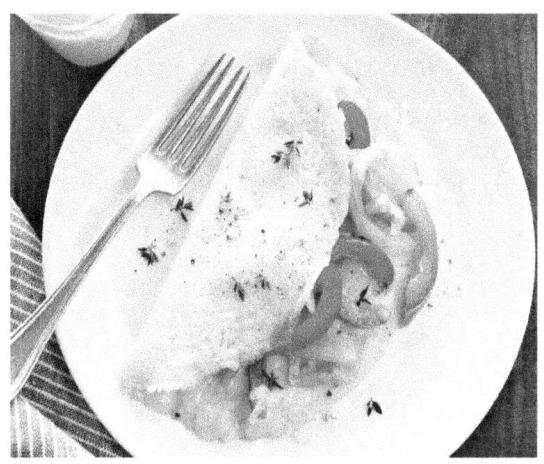

2. Western Omelet

INGREDIENTS:

Hen eggs - 6 pcs

Double cream or heavy sour cream - 2 tbsp.

Salt and pepper

Hard pressed cheese - 130 g

Butter - 56 g

½ yellow onion

½ green bell pepper

Diced ham - 150 g

METHOD OF PREPARATION

1. Blend eggs and cream (sour cream) until they are fluffy. Salt and pepper lightly.

2. Put 75 g of the finally grated hard pressed cheese and mix thoroughly.

3. Let the butter melt in a pan. Then add diced ham, finely chopped onion and pepper. Fry for 1-2 minutes. Add whipped eggs and fry again until ready.

4. Now minimise the temperature and cover the pan. Sprinkle finely grated cheese on top. Turn the omelet on a dish.

5. Serve hot with fresh green lettuce leaves and mild curry!

RECIPES OF KETO-DIET SALADS

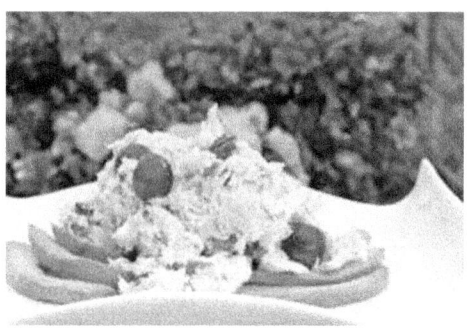

3. Chicken Salad with Soft Cream

INGREDIENTS:

Diced boiled chicken meat (or duck, turkey) - two glasses

Diced celery - 1/2 glass

Green onion rings - 1/2 glass

Ingredients for Lite Salad Dressing

Liquefied cream cheese - 85 gr.

Dried thyme - 1/2 teaspoon

Mayonnaise (better homemade) - 85 gr.

Dried tarragon - one teaspoon

Freshly ground pepper and salt

METHOD OF PREPARATION

1. Mix liquefied cream cheese and homemade mayonnaise, beat up this mass

2. Put the spices and beat again.

3. Add lite salad dressing to salad components and mix .

4. Add salt (pepper) to taste.

5. Roll up ready salad in green juicy lettuce leaves.

6. Enjoy your eating!

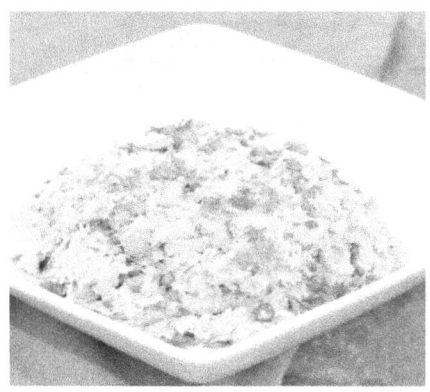

4. Tuna Salad with Capers

INGREDIENTS:

Tuna in olive oil - 1 can

Heavy sour cream - 50 g

Homemade mayonnaise - 180 g

Leeks - 3-5 pcs

Capers (or olives) - 1 tbsp

Chili flakes, to taste

Salt and pepper

METHOD OF PREPARATION

1. Drain the oil from canned.

2. Chop leeks.

2. Mix all components: tuna, sour cream, mayonnaise, leeks, capers and flavor with salt, black pepper or chili flakes (or hot chili sauce).

3. Serve with sesame crisp bread and boiled eggs.

NOTE! You may also cut eggs and add directly into the salad. It is tasty to use gherkins, olives instead of capers too.

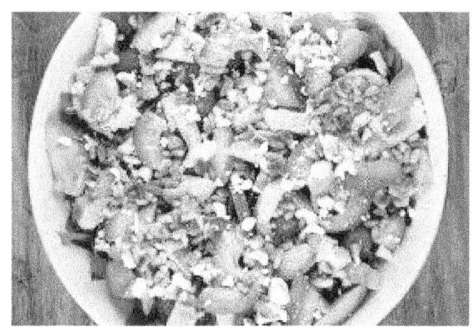

5. Goat-Cheese, Avocado and Bacon Salad

INGREDIENTS:

Goat cheese - 230 g

Bacon- 230 g

Avocados - 2 pcs

Walnuts - 115 g

Arugula lettuce - 115 g

Dressing

Fresh juice of ½ lemon

Homemade mayonnaise - 120 g

Olive oil - 120 g

Double cream - 50 g

METHOD OF PREPARATION

1. Before you start cooking this wonderful salad, switch on the oven and preheat it to 200°C . Place greaseproof paper in a shallow round cake pan.

2. Cut cheese into round slices (about 25 mm) and place in your round cake pan. Bake until golden crust.

3. Take bacon, slice it and fry until crispy.

4. Take an avocado wash it and dry with a paper towel, cut into small blocks.

5. Place arugula lettuce on the plate. On top of the leaves put the   avocado cubs, add the fried crispy bacon and round slices of fried goat cheese. Sprinkle with crushed walnuts.

6. Blend ingredients for a salad flavoring: freshly squeezed lemon juice, 120 g of olive oil, mayonnaise - 120 g and double cream - 50 g. Put a teaspoon of fresh herbs.

7. Salt and pepper to taste.

RECIPES OF DISHES FOR KETO-DIET DINNER (SUPPER)

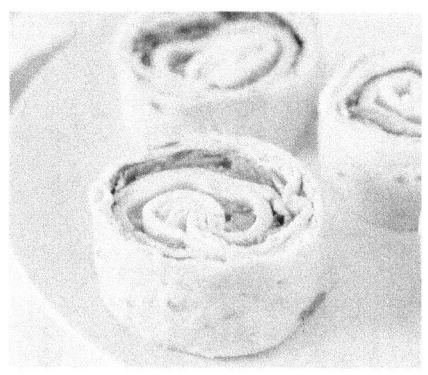

6. Turkey Rolls

INGREDIENTS:

Full-ream cheese - 230 g

Avocado - one piece

Light mayonnaise - one tablespoon

Garlic powder - ¼ tablespoon.

Baked turkey - 450 g

Lemon fresh

Bell pepper - one piece.

Cucumber - two pcs

METHOD OF PREPARATION

1. Soften full-cream cheese at room temperature. Turn it in a deep bowl and lightly beat up until creamy.

2. Carve the avocado in two, remove the pulpy substance. Use the fork and mash it, add one teaspoon of lemon juice. Put salt.

3. Slice cucumber and pepper.

4. Add garlic powder, mayonnaise and the flesh of the avocado to cheese. Mix all this mass for about a minute. Do a thick gravy.

5. Slice turkey meat. Spread meat slices with gravy on both sides, put one or two slices of pepper and cucumber.

6. Make turkey rolls.

7. Cauliflower Casserole in a Delicate Creamy Sauce

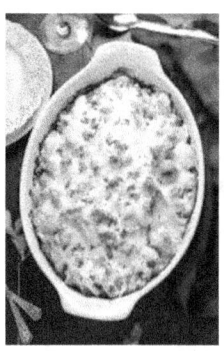

INGREDIENTS:

Fresh cauliflower - 900 g

White onion - 110 g

Butter - 1 tbsp

Cream cheese - 120 g

Heavy cream - 120 ml

Chicken broth - 60 ml

Grated cheese - 100 g

METHOD OF PREPARATION

1. Cut the cauliflower head into small curds. Put them in an enamel pan with lightly salt water and boil cook gently for 20-30 min, until cauliflower become soft and tender. Drain the vegetable and set aside. Or cook the cabbage in a steam cooker.

2. Take a deep pan and put 5 grams of butter. Let it melt. Then add sliced rings of white onion and cook it slowly — until it starts to color.

3.Then add to the fried onion cooked cauliflower. Mixing this mass with spatula, divide curds into smaller pieces. Now minimise the heat and cover the pan.

4. Turn mixture of chicken broth and cream into the pan. Then add cream cheese. Stir slowly ingredients until cheese is melted. You may pour a little more broth if pan's contents get thick. Finally, sprinkle everything with grated cheese. Mix once again.

5.Turn off a fire and shift fried cauliflower together with creamy sauce in a casserole pan, sprinkle finely grated cheese on the top of a dish.

6. Preheat oven to 150 degrees. Bake for 15-20 minutes.

7. Your cauliflower casserole in a delicate cream sauce is ready-to-serve!

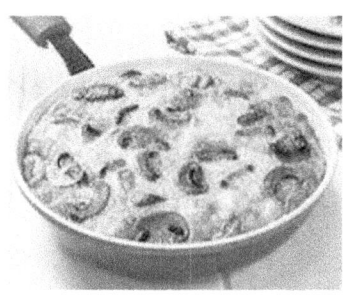

8. Mushroom and Cheese Frittata

INGREDIENTS FOR FRITTATA

Mushrooms - 455 g

Butter - 135 g

Scallions - 6 pcs

Fresh parsley - 1 tblsp

Fine salt - one teaspoon

Ground black pepper - 0,5 tsp

Fresh eggs - 10 pcs

Shredded cheese - 225 g

Mayonnaise - 250 g

Leafy greens - 115 g

INGREDIENTS FOR VINAIGGRETTE SAUCE

Olive oil - four tblsp

White wine vinegar - one tblsp

Salt - 0,5 tsp

Ground black pepper - ¼ teaspoon

METHOD OF PREPARATION

1. Heat up the oven to 175°. Mix together all components for vinaigrette sauce and set aside.

2. Slice, dice or chop the mushrooms.

3. Fry mushrooms in butter until golden (don't forget to mix). Minimize the heat.

4. Finely cut the scallions and combine it with fried mushrooms. Pepper and salt, put one tblsp of fresh green parsley.

5. Blend eggs, grated cheese, mayonnaise in an individual bowl. Put salt and pepper.

6. Grease baking bowl with a butter. Add the mixture of scallions and mushrooms then turn everything into it.

7. Bake about forty minutes or until our delicious frittata gets golden crust and begins pleasantly smell.

8. Cool slightly about 5 minutes and enjoy frittata with leafy green vegetables (eg. spinach) and the vinaigrette sauce.

RECIPES OF KETO-DIET BEVERAGES

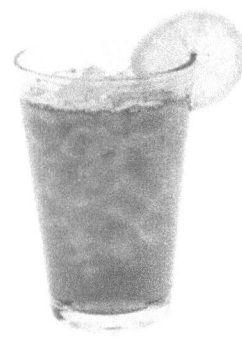

9. Ice Tea

INGREDIENTS:

Cool boiling water - 500 ml

Tea bag - 1 piece

Ice cubes - 1 glass

Slices of lemon, lime

Leaves of fresh mint - 5 pcs

METHOD OF PREPARATION

1. Put 1 tea bag of any type of tea (green, white, Yasmin or black), lemon, lime, wedges of orange, tangerine, peach, fresh mint leaves and 250 ml of cool boiling water in a big jug and put in the fridge. Cool about 60-120 minutes.

2. Get the tea bag, wedges of orange, tangerine, peach, slices of lime and green leaves out of the jug. At your wish, you may add variety of fresh flavoring.

3. Pour 250 ml of cool boiling water and serve with lots of cube ice.

4. Enjoy this wonderful tonic drink!

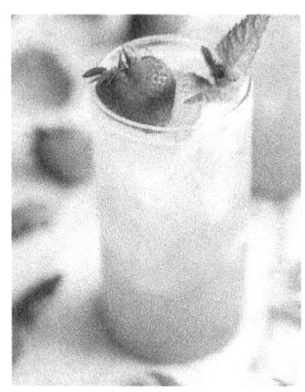

10. Strawberry Lemonade

INGREDIENTS:

Fresh strawberries - 303 g

Lemon juice - 244 g

Substitute for sugar - 200 g

Salt - 1 g

Cold boiling water - 710 g

METHOD OF PREPARATION

1. Take fresh berries, wash them and remove stems. Chop coarsely.

2. Puree the strawberries and other components (except water) in a liquidizer until completely smooth.

3. Turn the fruit puree to a pitcher and dilute with water.

4. Taste and make sweeter as necessary.

5. Mmmm!!! Yummy!!!

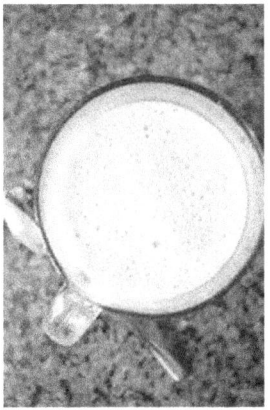

11. Dairy-Free Latte

INGREDIENTS:

Fresh eggs - 2 pcs

Coconut oil - 20 g

Boiled water - 1⅔ glasses

Vanilla extract - 1 pinch

Ground ginger - 10 g

METHOD OF PREPARATION

1. Blend all components together.

2. Enjoy immediately!

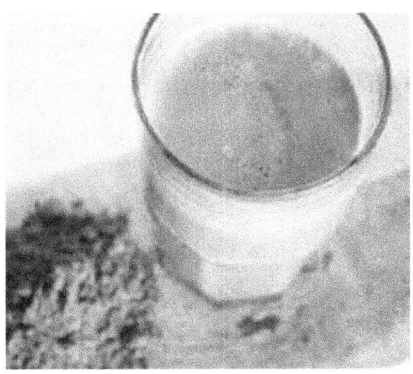

12. Protein Shake

INGREDIENTS:

Whey protein powder

Unsweetened almond milk – 227-453 g

METHOD OF PREPARATION

1. Mix required quantity of whey protein powder and almond milk in the blender bottle
2. If you like add double cream.
3. Ready to drink!

BY THE SAME AUTHOR

You are welcome to read another useful and very informative book by this author!

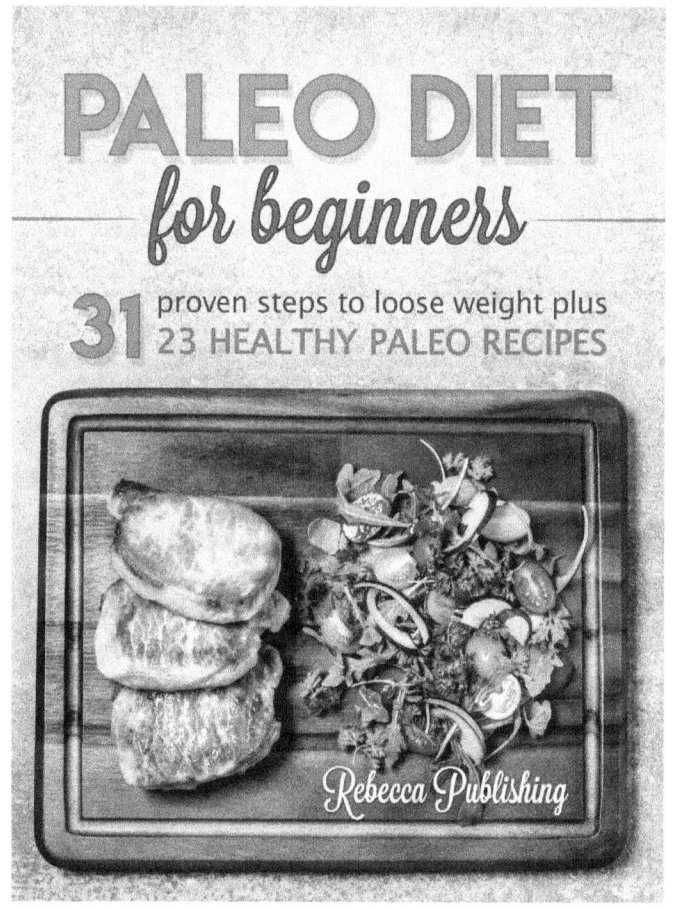

Please search this page over the www.amazon.com

www.amazon.com/s/ref=nb_sb_noss?url=search-alias%3Daps&field-keywords=B01MR9UU2O

www.ingramcontent.com/pod-product-compliance
Lightning Source LLC
Chambersburg PA
CBHW080830310526
45788CB00019B/2925